How to T

The Science

~y

Angelos Georgakis

www.livediversified.com

Table of Contents

Introduction

"Why would I need a book on how to take notes? Notes are just notes; they're not a big deal." "At the end of the day, everyone has their own way to take notes." "Anyway, no one taught me how to take notes in school or in college." "It comes naturally." "I feel like I always knew how to take notes! It's just notes. It's not rocket science!"

"Notes are just notes." **FALSE**. Scientists have found that note taking can be as mentally demanding as playing chess can be for an expert. While you take notes, you listen carefully to the lecturer, you process the new material, you organize it in your working memory, and you finally write down what you think is most important. All this happens while someone is talking at an average speed of three words per second and someone is writing it down at an average speed of one-third of a word per second. It doesn't sound easy now, does it?

Notes are an important tool for learning. We don't take notes just to record a few facts, so we can review them later. Learning happens as we take notes. Taking notes the right way leads to good study practices, better performance on exams, and long-term retention of information.

"It comes naturally." **FALSE**. Note taking is not obvious or intuitive. Research has shown that students fail to capture 40% of the main points in a typical lecture. First-year students capture only 11%. In some studies, even the best note takers seem to record less than 75% of the important information. People think they take good notes until they're told they don't. Few of us have consciously thought about how we take notes (let alone how to improve the quality of them). We

often reproduce the lecturer's phrases verbatim. We don't save time by systematic use of abbreviations. We fail to become a "good psychologist" of our lecturer. We fail to pick up his enthusiasm. We fail to interpret the tone of his voice. We fail to read his body language. And the result is that we fail to take good notes.

"Anyway, no one taught me how to take notes in school or in college." **TRUE**. Educators believe that students are able to assess the quality of their notes and follow good practices. However, studies have shown the exact opposite. The fact that there isn't a course in college dedicated to the art of taking notes (or learning in general) makes students believe that this is a natural skill that they can perfect with practice over the course of their studies.

"At the end of the day, everyone has their own way to take notes." **TRUE**. In this book, you may be surprised to learn that I don't make any reference to different types of note-taking systems like those that other books do. The reason is that it's the practices behind the note taking that matter most. For example, do not copy the lecturer's phrases word for word, but do generate main points in your own words. And you should leave space on your notes for adding comments and testing yourself later. I encourage students to use the Cornell note-taking system because it utilizes most of the principles of effective note taking. No matter which note-taking system you decide to follow, the cognitive effort you will have to expend is equally high.

Note taking may not be rocket science, but it's definitely science— cognitive science. And cognitive science has produced a lot of useful insights that we can use now to take better notes. This book presents these insights in simple words, so you can make the most of your notes and use them to study effectively.

At the end of every chapter, you will find notes with the main points. Basically, I took notes of my own book! :) These notes follow some good practices like abbreviation and paraphrasing. If you have any tips for me, please feel free to give me a shout at livediversified@gmail.com! Happy note-taking... or n/t! :)

The Note-taker's Manifesto

I have also created The Note-taker's Manifesto, a one-page PDF with all the good note-taking practices of this book! Download it, print it out, and stick it to the inside of your notebooks and remind yourself how you should take good notes.

You can download the NoteTaker's Manifesto by using this short link:

http://bit.ly/2zsmP9C

How to Learn More Effectively – Video Course Bonus

Here is the second bonus I promised to you – a mini video course on how to learn more effecively! You can get access to the course by using this short link: http://bit.ly/2ynIGPJ

In this course you'll learn:

- How to encode new information in your memory so you don't forget later.

- The truth about different learning styles according to research results

- How to solidify what you've learned using Recall Practice

- How to use Spaced Repetition to make the most of your learning results

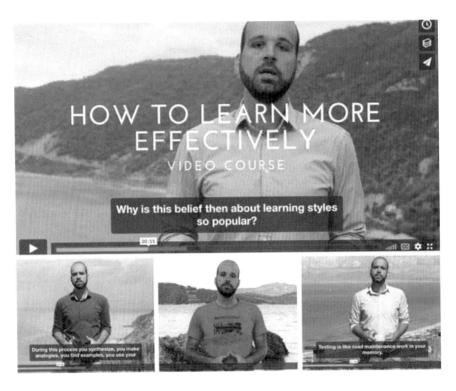

Get access to the course by using this short link: http://bit.ly/2ynIGPJ

Why bother taking notes?

When you take notes, actual learning is happening in your brain. Before you decide what's important to write down, you need to structure the information. You need to distinguish between key ideas and subordinate ones. This assumes though that you take notes properly and that you are not a transcribing machine, as we will explain later.

If you write something down, you are more likely to remember it later. Research has shown that those who take notes perform better on immediate and delayed tests of recall and synthesis than those who don't (see reference 1 in the References section). If you decide not to take notes, you may easily fall into a passive listening mode. On the contrary, note taking is a generative process that requires mental effort to capture the gist of what you listen to.

If you not only take notes but also review them, you are more likely to perform better on exams. Of course, this is the primary purpose of taking notes, i.e., to review and interact with them later. When you test yourself on the notes, when you elaborate by finding examples, or link them with previous notes, you end up learning effectively.

More importantly, studies have shown that reviewing self-produced notes leads to better recall than reviewing someone else's notes. When you review your own notes, you retrieve and strengthen information that *you* previously learned. When you review someone else's notes, it's the same as being exposed to something new for the first time.

Outside the class, research has shown that professionals who take notes are better problem solvers, make better decisions, and work better with others. For example, taking notes helps interviewers recall key facts about the applicants. Later, reviewing the notes leads to better judgement accuracy, i.e., selecting the best applicant.

Why Bother Taking Good Notes

During n/t, learning happens.

When you write sth down, you make it stick.

Better exam scores.

Best results -> review YOUR notes, not your friend's.

Good notes -> better prob solv'n and communication.

Do you think you take good notes?

If you think you take good notes, let's see what research studies have to say.

Students fail to capture 40% of the important points in a typical lecture (see reference 2 in the References section) while first-year students capture only 11% (see reference 3 in the References section). In some studies, even the best note takers recorded less than 75% of the important ideas. Students tend to record mostly information written on the blackboard while they capture only 10% of the information delivered orally (see reference 4 in the References section). Mistakes arise especially when it comes to equations, figures, diagrams etc. Surprisingly enough, when students spot an inaccuracy, most of the time they don't bother to correct their notes.

Students don't put much thought into coming up with a strategy to save time when taking notes. Hence, they make limited use of abbreviations, symbols, or diagrams that would allow them to focus more on the lecturer and record more important facts.

Studies have also shown that students don't pay attention to the lecturer's words as to what is important and what's not. For example, verbal expressions such as "first," "second," "third," "to sum up," "what's interesting here," "now we'll discuss," etc., often fail to ring a bell in the students' heads. In the same way, students fail to interpret the tone of voice of the lecturer, i.e., when he speaks with enthusiasm or emphasis.

Finally, students don't interact with their notes. They often read and reread their notes passively instead of forcing themselves to recall facts, elaborate, find examples, or link new information to already-known information. After class, they seldom space their learning practice by reviewing the notes often enough. Instead, they usually cram before an exam, compromising the long-term results of their learning.

Do you think you take good notes?

What research shows about students...

- Miss impt stuff.
- Make mistakes on charts, eqtn's.
- Lose time - dont use abbrev, symbols.
- Dont "read" the lecturer (impt words, voice, body lang).
- Dont interact w/t notes - Passive readers.
- Crammers - dont space their stud'n.

Why is it hard to take good notes?

The research findings of the previous chapter are so heartbreaking that it makes one wonder why we are so bad at taking notes. What makes note taking such a challenging task? To answer this question, we need to go a little deeper into how our memory works.

Note taking requires lots of cognitive effort. While you take notes, you need to listen carefully to what the instructor says, process the new material, organize the ideas into a structure (main ideas and sub-ideas), decide what's worth recording, and, finally, write it down. All this happens under severe pressure of time if you realize that an average speaker speaks at about three words per second, whereas the average student takes notes at one-third of a word per second. Hence, before you even manage to complete all the previous steps, the lecturer has already moved on to the next idea. To provide a comparison, scientists have found note taking to be as demanding as playing chess is for an expert in terms of cognitive effort (see reference 5 in the References section). In both skills, you need to retrieve information from your memory, construct a strategy, and then take action.

Note taking depends entirely on our working memory that is responsible for short-term storage and manipulation of information. When we take notes, our working memory is divided between two tasks: comprehension of new material and production of notes. The problem is that our working memory is limited in capacity and note takers struggle with finding the golden ratio between comprehension of information and recording of information.

On one hand, some students decide to devote all the power of their working memory to just write down what the professor says verbatim. However, this is not a good strategy, as the lecture becomes just a transcribing race with no learning happening. Instead of doing that, someone would clearly argue that it would be better to take someone else's notes or simply drop attendance and study on your own.

On the other hand, if you decide not to take notes at all, you will probably manage to understand more in the short term and score more on an immediate test. However, as we said earlier, students who take notes score better on delayed exams, especially if they review their notes. Hence, this is not a good strategy either.

Why is it hard to take good notes

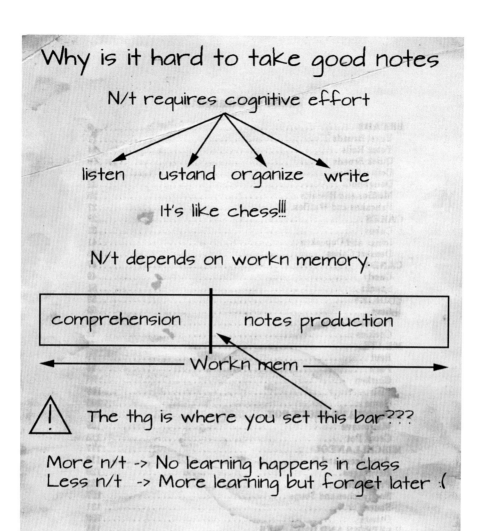

N/t requires cognitive effort

listen   ustand   organize   write

It's like chess‼️

N/t depends on workn memory.

| comprehension | notes production |

⟵ Workn mem ⟶

⚠️ The thg is where you set this bar???

More n/t -> No learning happens in class
Less n/t -> More learning but forget later :(

The secrets of taking good notes

Before the game

Prepare: Do some reading before taking notes. It will help you to pick up, understand, and organize the main points and content in the lecture. You will not only take better notes, but you will maximize your learning in class. Even if you spend just five minutes skimming through the lecture material, that will make a difference. Don't skip this part; it's crucial!

Watch a YouTube video before the class if you don't fancy reading: Okay, you don't feel like doing more reading today. Watch a short YouTube video about the subject you will be taking notes on tomorrow. I'm sure you can find a good video for anything on YouTube. Maybe there's a documentary, a tutorial, or an interview. For example, watch a historical documentary the night before the history class. That will increase your motivation and interest in the lecture. You will start making associations between the video and the lecture. You will be more absorbed into the lecture. This is when true learning happens.

Arrive early: Arrive to the class at least five minutes before the lecture starts. Take some deep breaths and relax. As we said, note taking is a very demanding cognitive process. This will not be a sleeping session. It will be a tough game. Spend some time doing some reading if you haven't done any earlier.

No matter whether you arrive early or late, sit in the first row: I never understand people who enter a room and always move towards the back. Note taking is hard. Why would you make it harder? You should be as close as possible to the lecturer and avoid distractions such as whispering or the noise in the back rows. Please don't get me started with arguments of the type: "I don't want to look like the professor's good boy," or "others will be looking at me," because I will refuse to comment.

During the game

Don't write everything down but don't leave too much out: First, you are not a voice recorder. Second, you will never be as good as a voice recorder. Third, there is no point in being a voice recorder. Make the most of the time you spend in a lecture. Try to learn as much as possible then and there. Don't spend all your working memory resources copying things onto your paper. Take notes in your own words and don't passively copy the lecturer's phrases verbatim. At the same time, make sure your notes are as complete as possible.

Beware of your "I knew-it-all-along" psychological bias: During a lecture, you will listen to something that sounds easy and logical. You might think: "That makes perfect sense, I could easily figure that out myself." When we are served with a fact, or the solution to a problem, everything makes sense. We feel that we could have easily arrived at the same fact or solution ourselves without any help. Don't fall into that trap. Test yourself on that dead-easy fact or solution later. And don't be surprised if you can't remember the fact or the solution.

Use the Cornell note-taking system (see link at the end of the book): This is a highly recommended note-taking system that requires and encourages an active approach from the note taker. Divide your sheets into two columns so the left-hand side takes about one-third of the sheet and the right-hand side takes up the remaining two-thirds of the sheet. Start taking down your notes in the right column. At the end of the lecture, complete the left column with keywords or questions for the respective notes in the right column. You may also leave some

17

space at the bottom to create a summary after the lecture. Below is a picture showing how you should "Cornell divide" your paper. There is also a very nice YouTube video (see link at the end of the book) that explains the Cornell notes.

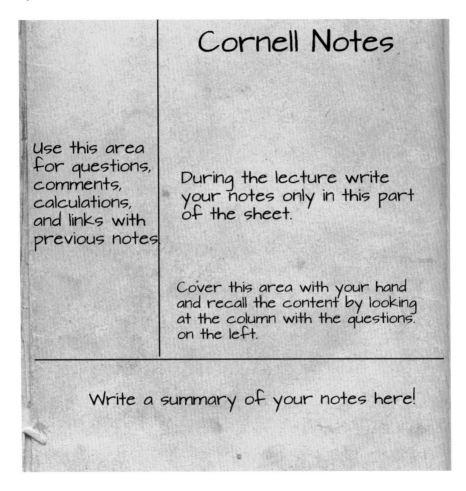

Cornell Notes

Use this area for questions, comments, calculations, and links with previous notes

During the lecture write your notes only in this part of the sheet.

Cover this area with your hand and recall the content by looking at the column with the questions. on the left.

Write a summary of your notes here!

If you don't like the Cornell notes, make sure you leave enough space for later: You should interact with your notes. Once you take them, you will review them a lot. Hence, you will need extra space to elaborate, provide examples, write down questions, and complete your notes in case you missed something.

Abbreviate: Every subject has words that can be abbreviated and easily recognized. If you're taking notes on crime and punishment, I would bet all those *D*'s probably stand for Dostoyevsky. Use shorthand symbols like **w/** for *with*, **w/o** for *without*, **C19** for *nineteenth century,* etc. You can find a nice resource with abbreviations at the end of the book (see link at the end of the book). Develop your own abbreviations that make better sense to you.

Listen for particular words: Words like "what's important here," "an interesting fact is," the main idea here," etc. should definitely trigger a note-taking event. Also, listen for introductory and concluding phrases such as "the next topic will be …," "to sum up," "to recap," or phrases that help you organize the material such as "first," "second," or "third." Most of the important things are said either in the very beginning or in the very end of the lecture. Hence, don't be the last to arrive and don't be the first to shoot off.

"Read" your lecturer with all your senses: Pay attention to the lecturer's tone of voice and body language. For example, he may raise his hand, or speak slowly to highlight something important. That is when you should definitely be taking notes. If he speaks very quickly, he probably wants to skip something trivial and move on to something more important. Watch out for moments when he becomes enthusiastic, or adds emphasis to something. Make sure you record that something.

After the game

Recap and complete any missing bits: Spend five minutes right after the lecture to complete any missing information. Make sure you understand all the abbreviations. You may have to write out full words for some of them that might be unclear later. Fill the left column of your notes if you're using the Cornell notes system. Elaborate, find examples, and focus again on the main ideas.

Compare your notes with your buddies' notes: Compare your notes with those of your peers and spot errors. Pay particular attention to graphs, formulas, and mathematical equations. Research has shown that students make the most mistakes on those. A great thing to do is to establish a group of two to three friends and check each other's notes at the end of the lecture. Your friend may have spotted something important that you missed and vice versa. From experience, I know that this collective power in college can do wonders.

Review your notes on the same day: As most of the forgetting happens within the first few hours, it's very important to review your notes on the same day. Below you can see the forgetting curve that shows how quickly we forget after the first exposure to new information. A few reviews early on will make this curve more flat and new information more durable from forgetting.

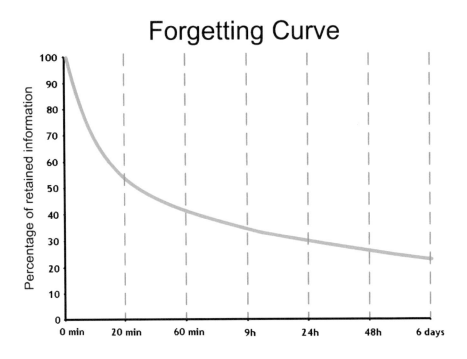

Review your notes after a good sleep: It has been shown that sleep plays an important role in the consolidation of new information in our long-term memory. While we sleep, new memories are strengthened and reorganized. Hence, review your notes again the next day or the day after.

Review should be hard: When I say "review your notes," I don't mean you should passively look over your notes a couple of times. When I review my notes, I test myself on the new information. I cover the right column of my Cornell notes and practice retrieval. I squeeze my mind to remember. I link the new information to information I already know. I make associations. I find examples. I write down questions to follow up on at the next lecture. The harder you make your learning, the more effective and durable it becomes.

Use Cal Newport's technique of active recall: Cal Newport is an assistant professor of computer science at Georgetown University and author of the popular blog Study Hacks (http://calnewport.com/blog/). Cal says that if you find yourself spending hours silently reading and highlighting your notes, you are certainly doing the wrong thing. Instead, leave your notes aside, and try to explain out loud whatever you're trying to learn as if you were explaining it to someone else. This process is strenuous, but this is the only way to make the most of your learning. We can compare learning to a gym workout. If you want to see results in the gym, you should make your workout hard and push yourself with those last two killing reps. The same happens with learning. If you decide to cheat and avoid testing, you don't make the information secure from long-term forgetting.

Review your notes regularly thereafter: We take notes, so we interact with them regularly. Studies have shown that spaced practice is the key to effective learning. By testing yourself at spaced intervals and allowing a little bit of forgetting to happen, retrieval pathways are strengthened and retrieval becomes easier in the future. So, it's a good practice to review your notes regularly. For example, review the week's notes on the weekend. Then, review them again every two weeks or every month.

Never, never, never cram: Cramming is a common student practice before an exam. Okay, I will have to admit something. If you have only one day to review your notes before an exam, maybe cramming is better than spaced study sessions. However, if your goal is to retain the information for a longer period, or you have a more advanced course on the same subject in the future, cramming is the most inefficient way to study. You may feel you learn so much in a short time, but what you don't see is that the rapid learning gains will soon become rapid forgetting losses. Promise you will never cram again.

Beware of your "will-know-it-all-along" psychological bias: Cramming and rereading produce a false illusion of mastery. You feel overconfident that you know the new material and that you will remember it forever ("will-know-it-all-along" or foresight bias). Research has shown, though, that we are poor judges of our future performances based on our current performances. This is the reason we should test ourselves on our notes at different points in time to solidify new information.

Evaluate your notes: You should always go back to your notes and evaluate them. Does the way you take notes help you to study? Do you make mistakes? Do you capture the main points that come up on the exams? You are encouraged to discuss and show your notes to the instructor of the course and ask for advice.

Review your notes during an exam-free period: In the summertime when you don't have any classes, you should review what you have learned over the semesters. It's only then, when you have successfully passed all of your exams, that you have no stress. In that state of calmness, learning becomes more effective. That consolidation of knowledge will make a difference over the next semester in recalling previously learned material and linking it with new material.

Secrets of N/t

Before
Prepare: Preread syllabus - Make most of lec - even 5min OK
Youtube: Short video - get idea of lec topic -> motivation
Arrive early: Preread, breathe, relax.
Sit 1st row: To listen better, no noise, no distractions

During
Too much is less : Can't write down everything - but dont miss a lot.
Knew-it-all-along bias: Test your self even on thgs that sound "logical".
Cornell notes: Left: questions, Right: Your notes, Bottom: Summary
If not Cornell: Leave space for commts, additions, questions
Abbreviate: Make words shorter, save time, eg without = w/o.
N/t trigger words: "What's impt..." "Main idea is..." or "1st, 2nd, 3rd..."
"Read" lecturer: Voice speed, body lang, emphasis, enthusiasm

After
Complete notes: Missing stuff, abbrev's, Cornell left colmn
Compare notes: Check w/ friends, esp. formulas, eqn's - make team
Same day review: Review soon - forgetting happens early
Review after sleep: New info gets reorganized while we sleep
Review hard: No passive review - TEST - engage - link - elaborate
Active recall: Explain out loud new info as if ur teacher -no cheating
Review often: (same notes) using testing - weekly, monthly etc.
No cramming: Space studying for long-term results
Will-know-it-all-along: (bias) Dont be sure you'll remember tomorrow...
Evaluate notes: Effective? Mistakes? Main pnts? Ask instructor
Summer review: Review notes when stress-free - better retention

Note-taking tips from two gurus

Successful people are good note takers. To pump you with more motivation, I decided to present some of the note-taking practices of two gurus of the sport. The first is probably the most famous inventor of all times, Thomas Edison, the man who invented the light bulb. The second is Tim Ferriss, a contemporary learning fanatic and author of the international best-selling book *The 4-Hour Workweek* (see link at the end of the book).

Thomas Edison

Thomas Edison certainly loved taking notes. His diary contains over 5,000,000 pages of notes and is stored in the United States' National Archives. Edison was obsessed with recording any important piece of information that he came across while conducting his experiments. It saved a lot of time and effort from repeating the same experiments unnecessarily.

It was obviously time consuming to go through thousands of papers looking for a single document. For this reason, he created an efficient system of archiving his records based on chronological order and subject. He created numerous groupings, files, folders, etc. which helped him to get to the right piece of information in a reasonably short time.

His notes also proved valuable when he had to defend himself against competitors over a patent (the man had 1,093 U.S. patents in his name). Edison was victorious in the lawsuits, as his competitors couldn't compete with his thoroughly written proof.

To answer to **what, where, when, why, and how much** was easy for any aspect of work Edison was involved in when reading his notes. These details accompanied every financial record. He also kept records of all the incoming and outgoing correspondence. You can imagine how difficult that was at a time when photocopy machines did not exist.

The act of writing something down helps long-term recall. Even if Edison couldn't recall a specific detail when he was asked about something, he could still remember that he had recorded it. By searching his notes, he would quickly come up with the information he was looking for. Note takers often have this feeling when they know they have recorded something ("Just let me look at my notes!") Hence, if you want to remember it, write it down!

Tim Ferriss

The main purpose of taking notes is to review them later. Tim Ferriss keeps tons of notes in his notebooks and has found a great way to refer back to them quickly using an indexing system:

1. Number every right-hand page of your notebook but not the left (e.g., 1, 2, 3, etc.).

2. Whenever you complete a page, put the page number in an index on the inside cover (front or back) and a few words to describe the content.

3. If the information is on the left-hand side of the page add ".5" to the page number in the index. For example, if you are writing on the page marked "10" (you see the number on that page) and you flip it over, whatever you write at the back of the page should have "10.5" in the index.

I have been using this indexing system for myself, and I have come to realize that its beauty has not only to do with indexing and quick referencing but with another important purpose. Because you have to write a few things about the content in the index, you need to review your notes. This isn't just a passive copy, as you need to understand what's important there, organize and filter the main ideas, and write a brief description in the index. Hence, by using this system, you not only get the benefit of indexing but you are also forced to do good reviews of your notes.

Tim also gives some useful advice on choosing the right kind of notepad depending on the situation. Hence, a big notepad is great for taking notes for a book or an article, and generally more lengthy projects when you don't want to flip the pages continually trying to find what you want. A hard-backed rectangular notebook—the small, handy one that can easily fit in the back pocket of your jeans—comes in handy when you need to jot down points during a phone interview, telephone numbers, to-do lists, and any ideas that may come on the fly while you're on the move. You can find a link to more of Tim's tips at the end of the book.

Tips from 2 gurus

Thomas Edison

Fanatic note-taker   Notes < keep you organized / save you time

Organise notes by date/content

Notes -> document of proof (he used notes agst
            competitors to prove patent ownership)
      -> long-term recall (even if you forget, you
            remember it's in your notes...)

Tim Ferriss

Indexing System

1) Find info quickly
2) Chance to review
when you fill index

Inside Cover (index)
10:    Working Memry
10.5: Memory cells
11:    Main pnts
11.5: Main pnts

Working Memory	10
At the back of this page -> 10.5 (no need to write... you know...)	

Big notebook: long projects (book, blog articles etc.)
Small one: jot down ideas wherever your are

Pen and paper versus the computer

With more and more students taking notes on their laptops in the classroom, note takers are raising the question whether we should take notes by hand or switch to electronic note taking. As with many aspects in life, there are pros and cons involved with both ways. However, can we announce a winner?

The ones who use laptops can certainly produce more notes, which gives them an advantage. As we mentioned earlier, research has shown that those who record more facts during the lecture score better on delayed tests. Laptop fans also mention the technical advantages. For example, their electronic notes are easily synchronized and automatically saved using "cloud applications" (Google Drive, Evernote), eliminating the risk of losing them. Also, the notes are accessible to review any time from any computer connected to the Internet.

However, the laptop note takers are more prone to transcribing word for word what the lecturer says. Hence, they devote more of their working memory power to transcription rather than comprehension. On the contrary, longhand note takers, as they are unable to write everything down, spend time to understand and filter the most important information that deserves to be recorded. As far as the technical advantages are concerned, their answer is that pen and paper, first, don't need to be recharged, and second, are distraction-free (no email, no Facebook, etc.).

A recent study (see link at the end of the book) proves that taking notes by hand promotes long-term recall. In this study, sixty-five college students were divided into two groups (pen and paper, laptop). The two groups were asked to watch a *TED Talks* show—on an interesting but not very well known topic—and take notes. Laptops were obviously disconnected from the Internet.

In the end, the two groups were asked to answer factual-recall questions as well as conceptual-application questions based on what they watched. The researchers found that although both groups performed well on recalling facts, the longhand note takers performed better on conceptual questions.

The laptop note takers produced more verbatim notes compared with the handwritten note takers. Overall, the students who produced more notes and the students who did not take word-for-word notes performed better on the test. Hence, the laptop advantage of producing more notes was cancelled out by more verbatim overlap. Interestingly enough, even when the researchers encouraged the laptop users to produce notes in their own words, they still had more verbatim overlap than longhand note takers.

The researchers also found that longhand note takers scored better on recall tests one week later when participants were given a chance to review their notes before taking the test. Once again, the amount of verbatim overlap was associated with worse performance on conceptual items.

Another study (see link at the end of the book) that used advanced techniques like electromagnetic resonance has shown that handwriting activates regions of the brain associated with thinking, language, and memory. Handwriting practice helps with learning letters and shapes, can improve idea composition and expression, and may aid fine motor-skill development. Researchers found that adults studying new symbols, such as Chinese characters, might enhance recognition by writing the characters by hand. Some physicians say handwriting could be a good cognitive exercise for those who want to keep their minds sharp as they age.

On the basis of all of the above, and not because I personally take notes by hand, going old-school on note taking is a good, solid plan.

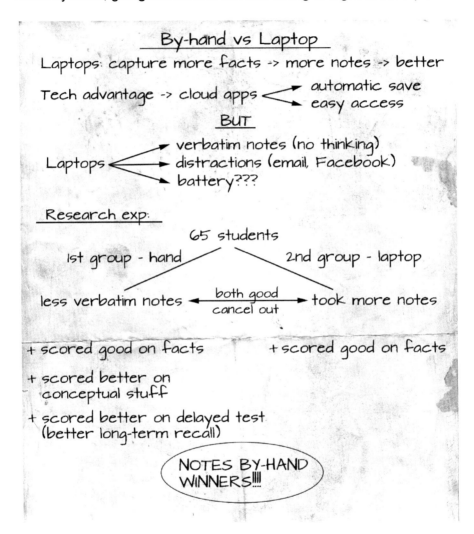

People these days tend to over-rely on technology and use computers for just about everything. They have forgotten to use pen and paper and fail to see it as the best option to take notes.

As we know, computers can cost anywhere between $500 and $1,000 and then you have to take account of the additional cost of maintenance. You can opt for good old pen and paper as these are the best tools that you can use to take down notes.

To further convince you, here is an analysis of using computers and pen and paper.

Computers

Computers are smart little devices that are extensively popular around the world. They leave us with a variety of uses such as providing entertainment, accessing websites, learning opportunities, socializing, etc.

There may be countless benefits to using a computer to perform mundane tasks. In fact, it is also quite easy to carry your laptop around and use it whenever you want to. It is primarily a boon for students who can whip it out in the classroom and take down notes. And it's not just students who love it but also lecturers who like to switch it on as soon as they enter the classroom and showcase lessons on PPTs.

Now all this might sound great and convenient. However, it is not as convenient as you may think as there are many issues related to using computers to take notes. To begin with, it is not possible for everybody to type at the same speed. What if some of the students are slow at typing and miss out on taking down some important notes? It might cause them to be left behind.

Another issue associated with computers is that it can lead to unnecessary distractions. Once the computer is in front of you, you will feel like surfing the Internet, looking things up, etc. You might think about accessing social media, visiting online stores, etc. All this can take away focus from the work at hand.

Some believe taking down notes using the computer will not make you an active learner and leave you as a passive one. This can impact your thinking capacity and make you pay less attention to whatever is being said.

By replacing your laptop with pen and paper, you can write down more and take meaningful notes. In fact, there is no comparison between the two as writing manually makes you think more about the content of what you are writing.

When you take it down manually and realize that the lecturer is going too fast, then your alert mind will make you take down only those notes that are important and essential to keep you ahead of others. In fact, it can help you retain the information for longer as you tend to pay more attention while writing something down as compared to typing it.

When a person types on a computer, the subconscious mind kicks in and the person is unable to know where his fingers are landing. This can make it a bit difficult for people to focus on the task and remain distracted. This is not the case when you take notes down using a pen and paper, as you will know exactly what you are writing. You will be engaged in knowing what you are taking down and focus on the lecturer's words instead of the mechanics of typing.

As per a study conducted on writing versus using the computer to take notes, it was found that students who wrote down their notes using the traditional method of pen and paper did much better than those who used a computer to take down the notes. This is because the students paid more attention while taking the notes down in written format.

Using laptop

Although we spoke about the computer not being a good choice to take down notes, it is understood that many still prefer to use it to take notes. After all, they will have spent quite a lot of money on the laptop and will want to put it to good use. For this, here are some tips to bear in mind that will help you make the most of your computer's ability in taking notes.

If you happen to be one of those who can type super fast but cannot write fast enough, then you can use your laptop to take down all the notes. Make sure you type fast and take down all that your professor says. Once you go home, go through all the writing and skim all the essential parts. Write down the important elements in your notebook.

That way, you can revise and learn as you will take the information down twice. You can also take out printouts of the notes and highlight just the important bits if you do not wish to take notes twice. This will also allow you to go over all the notes again and revise your copy. You can also add in extra notes and side notes and attach them to the papers.

In the case of having missed out on taking down something, then contact your professor to ask if he can email a copy of the notes to you. You can modify the email and mark the critical parts and take a print out. You can also collect the slides if your professor does not need them anymore.

If you still do not like the concept of taking notes using a laptop and would like to do it the traditional way, then you can make use of a tablet. You can use a stylus as a pen to write down the notes in your tablet's notepad. You can also simply use your finger to write. The advantage of this is that you can take down diagrams as well. You can draw the diagrams as you work and make it a visually appealing note that helps you recall information easily.

Making use of pen and paper

You will have by now understood that using a computer is not necessarily the best way to take notes as it does not feel the same as taking notes manually. But we looked at some ways in which you can get around the issue and use your computer. In this segment, we will look at the use of pen and paper to take notes and some issues related to this method.

It is a myth that it is only the previous generation who were interested in making use of pen and paper to take notes and the younger generation is disinterested. Many youngsters still prefer to make use of pen and paper to take down notes. But there is one disadvantage associated with taking notes the traditional way. As you know, not everybody will be able to write as fast as others and may end up missing out on some critical notes. It can bring on stress, as people hold the fear of missing out on valuable information. They might also start writing at a superfast speed, which can lead to pain in the hands from repetitive actions.

To get around this issue, you can engage in selective writing. As per this technique, you write down only the important aspects of the data and let go of unnecessary words. These can be vowels, joining words and other such parts that can be eliminated from the sentence without impacting it. For example, you can shorten:

"Early to bed and early to rise, makes a man healthy, wealthy and wise" will be changed to 'Early to bed, early to rise > healthy and wise'. It might not look like a complete sentence but will be good enough to tell you what the sentence is trying to imply.

Another issue associated with writing vs. typing is that some people tend to have horrible handwriting. In fact, their writing will be so bad that they will not be able to understand it themselves. In such a case, the trick will be to write more often and write slowly. This will help you practice more and work on enhancing your handwriting. Take an hour's time every day to write sentences that cover all the alphabets in English.

Write it fast and write it slowly. One of the best sentences to practice with is "The quick brown dog jumped over the lazy fox." This has all the letters in the English alphabet and can be used to improve handwriting.

The advantages associated with writing are many. You can practice your handwriting, revise more, understand the concepts in a better way, develop the habit of taking down more notes, etc. All these can help you improve your writing prowess and learn more.

You can come up with a method of your own to take down notes. You do not have to follow others or their advice. Do what works for you. The best thing to do will be to try out both typing and handwritten notes and choose the one that suits you the best.

Importance of taking notes

There are many advantages associated with taking down notes as compared to borrowing them. Many would consider it redundant and useless, especially those who are used to borrowing the notes from their professors. They will not be exposed to taking down the notes and rely on the material provided by the professor.

However, those notes might not be comprehensive and leave out specific details. In such a case, it would be best to take down your notes so that you can mention all the essential aspects and not leave anything out.

Most professors will only write down the heading of the topics and a subtopic or two and start explaining about it. These will be pretty much useless as the student cannot learn just the headings and pass exams. He should be exposed to the content as well so that he can learn more and do better. So even if you manage to get the professor's notes, you will not be able to do justice to the topic. In such a case, it is best to take down the notes yourself, and some reasons are as follows.

As you might be aware, there is a plethora of reasons that make note-taking a good idea. In fact, there are just so many that explaining all will take us a day or two. So, to keep you motivated into taking notes, here are a few of the important reasons.

The very first advantage associated with taking notes is that it can help you focus on what you are writing. As per study reports, those who pay attention while writing can extend the same towards other fields of their life. Right from the time when people hold the pen in their hands to the time they place the last full stop (or period), taking notes requires extreme concentration. So, they will be able to focus on various other aspects as well including work, socializing, etc. The subconscious mind is altered making it easier for people to concentrate and focus on different actions and routines. Therefore, the more you write, the more practice and knowledge you gain.

When you take down notes, you tend to be part of an active learning environment. You can easily write down all the information and highlight the main aspects of the topic. This can help you prioritize your basic skills and help you to improve your overall confidence and concentration.

When you make the effort of engaging in selective learning, then you choose only the essential bits of the topic and do away with the unnecessary parts. This prioritizing can help you save time and effort and make you achieve more. It can also help you get over stress and develop a peaceful mind.

Writing and typing also aids in enhancing your vocabulary and increasing your creative writing skills. These two happen to be two very important aspects of learning. You have to try and make use of as many different words and sentences to ensure that you dig deep into understanding the different ways in which you can form and structure sentences and make the most of your note taking activity.

One aspect of taking notes that makes it a useful activity is that you can work on re-wording sentences and make the topic your own. It helps in improving your overall writing skills and gives you the confidence to write more. As and when you start taking note-taking seriously, you increase your confidence levels and become more and more skillful at writing. Your speed will improve drastically, and you will be able to speak out more freely. You will not refrain from addressing your crowd when your professor calls you up to give a lecture.

One aspect of taking notes is organizing. You have to organize the information in an orderly fashion so that it is easier for you to read and learn faster. You can make use of bullet points to write down the information and organize it in a way that is easy to follow.

When you take down notes, you have the chance to enhance your attention span. The human attention span lasts for 12 seconds and can get lower owing to the exposure to television and laptops. According to scientists, the human attention span is less than that of goldfish. This means that we are unable to focus on any one thing for more than a few seconds. In such a case, you have to make it a point to write more so that you can increase your concentration level. This can help you enhance your productivity and do more with your time and effort.

It is believed that taking notes can help you increase your attention span to between 30 minutes to 1 hour. This is quite a drastic time frame considering most of us are unable to concentrate for more than a minute. The more you write, the more your concentration level improves.

Tips to take down notes

One of the main advantages of taking down notes is that you can always have reference points. This is one of the most important aspects associated with taking notes and making the most of your habit. It is especially useful for history students who must learn a lot. It is not easy or practical to keep everything in your mind. You have to move around from class to class, and this can take a toll on your concentration. You might end up feeling disorientated in class and miss out on details.

So, to prevent this, you must make it a point to take down notes during every class. That way, you can feel happy knowing that you have all the notes to refer to and can pull them up any time. You do not have to rework on taking notes to revise. You will feel good knowing that your work has been cut in half and you can do more in your spare time.

Here are some simple ways in which you can prepare yourself to take down notes during class.

First off, you must be prepared for it. Ensure that you carry everything that you will need to take down the notes. This includes your books, notepads, pens, pencils, erasers, markers, etc. All these will be used to take down the information that is being shared in class. Be prepared for the class and know in advance what will be taught. For example, if it's a math class, then chances are you will require graphs and geometry set to make diagrams and graphs. Prepare these and carry some pencils and highlighters so that you can make the necessary drawings. Have the tools you need for the subject.

Next up, you must increase your skills at paying attention to whatever is being said in class. Without paying attention, you will not be able to take down the notes accurately. It is quite difficult to take something down without knowing what the professor is speaking about. If you find your mind is being distracted, then it will be next to impossible to make a note of the information that is being communicated.

Bear in mind that education is not cheap and your parents will have spent quite a lot of money on educating you. In such a case, you must do justice to all the money that has been spent and make the most of your classes.

The education you receive in school and college is the most important of all. You will be using it all through your life, especially when taking up a job. All this is not meant to stress you out but, instead, help you realize the value of education and how taking notes can help you make the most of your abilities.

When you pay attention in class, you not only put yourself in a better position to hold on to the information for life but also be able to use it practically. So instead of sitting in class not paying attention or doing important things, you can instead shift focus to taking down notes and recording all the information you need. Paying attention to whatever is being said in class can not only help you reproduce it better but also act upon it and use it in your everyday life.

Another aspect that you can consider is taking notes using different techniques. It is understood that it can get a bit monotonous taking notes in the same way, every day. To prevent this monotony, you can try taking up different methods of note-taking to make the most of your habit. Once you find the right technique, you can make use of it to increase your overall potential in taking notes and remembering things for longer.

You will have to make it a point to make it as easy as possible for you to take down notes during class as you will not have too much time on your hands. For your convenience, you can write down the headings and subheadings so that you can easily start filling in the information as the class progresses. You can also add footnotes so that you record any vital information that you can refer back to when you look back at your notes.

Order is everything so make sure you place all the information in an orderly fashion. You should be able to go to the desired page and paragraph without putting in much effort.

Make it a point to use colored markers so that you can mark the important information.

If you wish to use the computer to take notes, then make sure you have your notepad open so that you can record all the information during class. You can make use of the tips mentioned in the previous chapter to make it easier for yourself to record the data and retrieve it as and when you want it.

Here too, you have to prepare for class by mentioning the headings, subheadings, titles and footnotes. These will help you keep things organized and help you record information faster.

Develop the habit of editing your notes within 24 hours of taking them down so that you are prepared for your next class. Dedicate an hour or two every day so that you can record all the information and have enough time to go over it again. Try your best to read and revise the data then and there while your memory of the information in class is fresh.

As you can see, there are many things that you can do as students to make the most of your note taking habits.

Ryan Holding, Maria Popov and Robert Greene

In a bit, we will look at some simple note taking methods that you can employ to make it easier to take down notes.

But before that, we will look at some note taking experts and the skills they make use of to take down notes efficiently and in express time. These experts have developed the habit over several years and have perfected their methods through regular practice. You too can look up to their practices as a source of inspiration to take down notes.

Ryan Holiday: The Note Card System

Ryan Holiday is a note taking expert who has designed a system using index cards and files that help you organize data and plan your assignments and papers. Although he says that this system might not work for all, there is evidence that says the system is suitable for everyone.

This system includes taking down ideas and concepts on an index card. It can be a single word, a long sentence or just a small para. It is up to you to decide what to add to the index card. You can use these as cue cards to prompt you and remember something easily.

According to Ryan Holiday, this is not the best method to use for those who wish to organize all the information and require in-depth notes. However, this is not true. It is ideal for all students as they can easily learn a concept by writing down keywords that will prompt them to remember something easily.

This method is easy to follow. All you have to do is write down the ideas and concepts on an index card. It can be just a simple word, a sentence or a small paragraph. These can be treated as ideas, concepts and quotes that you can refer to, to remember a concept. As soon as you see a word, you will immediately remember the concept that is related to it. These keywords can be written down to your liking so that it is easier to remember the notes.

According to Holiday, it is a great idea to make use of this technique as it helps you in separating the wheat from the shaft. In other words, it helps you remember only those things that are important and do away with the rest. With time, you will see that it is easy to use this method and make the most of it remember and recall things better.

Once you listen to the piece of information, you have to wait for a little time before transferring the information to the cards. In this time, you should think of all the keywords that you would put down on the cards and which ones will make it easier for you to remember the concepts.

According to Holiday, it is best to write down the words on the top right-hand corner of the cards. This makes it easier to find the right word while going through the different cards.

If you happen to have many themes to go through, then you must make use of duplicate cards. These cards can help you make the most of your note taking skills and ensure that you recall things easily.

This type of system is especially useful for students. It can help them organize the information in a systematic manner and be of great use while studying. The themes, information, meaning and other aspects of the reading material can be easily recorded on the index cards and pulled out when needed to go through the study material.

Students will find it easier to carry the cue cards to class as compared to books. They can carry more cards, write down more and make a note of all the important data on the cards. However, one complaint that some students tend to have with this method is that it can be a little time-consuming. Holiday too has himself stated that it could be a little time consuming and not ideal for all students. It can prove to be a little tedious and tire students out faster.

Therefore, he suggests that this method should be used for close reading so that it helps students finish their assignments faster. The themes and concepts that are recorded on the cards can be used to study faster and revise easily.

Robert Greene is a well-known author who taught his note taking habits to Holiday. Robert Greene was known for introducing the note card system. In fact, if you now Google his name then you will find many search results suggesting the same.

As the system began to gain popularity, many modifications were introduced. These modifications including writing down the connections and the theme of the information on the index cards on the right-hand side. Some then began to write down the characteristics, the traits and the overall moods of the theme. This makes it easier to recall the data and understand the concept easily.

The system is quite adaptable and can be modified to your liking. This makes it one of the most preferred systems, as it is flexible. You can record more and ensure that you increase your overall learning capacity.

This system need not be limited to use by students alone and can also be adopted by people in the army, navy, armed forces, people in IT jobs, office goers, etc. It will be easier for them to take down notes and refer back to them as and when they like. They also do not have to carry around heavy books and can carry just the small cards to record the information on top.

Maria Popova

Maria Popova is a famous Bulgarian blogger who is well known for her book called Brain Pickings. The book is not her only work as she has written many articles in papers such as New York Times and the Harvard Journal and also maintained a successful blog.

Apart from these, she has also written extensively about the learning systems that she developed from an early age. She has outlined the different methods that she believes help people learn and hold on to information at a faster rate and recall it quicker.

The technique she employs makes use of remembering as much as you can so that you can recall all the information faster. This is especially useful if you record the data on the index cards. For example, you have to read a book for your English class and write a report on it. For this, you can find the essential themes of the text and highlight them first. This is done so that it is easier to go about preparing the report with a framework in place. So the first rule would be to outline the important bits and make sure that you highlight those using bold colors so that your attention goes to the main points when you wish to revise.

Popova advises that you use an index at the very beginning or the end of the book. This should include the outline of the book along with the main points that happened in the book. This will give you a quick reference point and make it easier to record the other information. As and when you go about reading the book, you will find it easier to highlight the important bits and make a note of the points that are important. You can keep adding in all the important points as and when you go about reading the book. This method makes it extremely easy for you to refer back to the content as and when you like.

By now it might look like taking notes is a bit more than active reading and that happens to be a good way of looking at it. While taking notes, all your focus is on highlighting and jotting down the important parts of the book. This makes it easier for you to focus on the content and increase your knowledge on the subject. This helps you build knowledge and makes it easier for you to revise.

With active engaging in note taking, you increase your chances of remembering as much as you can so that it is easier to recall it later. This, therefore, makes the very basis of Popova's technique.

One other point that Popova brings up is that it is best to create symbols, acronyms and such visual aids that will make it easier for you to remember things for longer. It can help you remember better and longer. I'm sure you have heard in school and other places that graphs and drawings help you remember more. Therefore, draw and sketch more so that you can remember the information for longer.

Acronyms are your best weapon when it comes to remembering things for longer periods of time. You can make acronyms for the syllabus so that you can easily recollect the information. For example, go through some mnemonics to get an understanding of how it works. Once you start doing it, you will be more confident in it.

Popova advises that people make use of pencils to highlight in their books and not markers. It will be easier to erase in case you make mistakes, and the book will look neater.

So, to say the least, this type of learning can help you get a grasp of whatever you are reading. You can retain the information longer and make sense of it when you look back at it.

The downside associated with this system is the setup. You might have to spend quite some time looking for information that you wish to record and highlight. This can prove to be quite a tedious task and one that makes you change your mind about taking up this particular method.

You might sometimes have to record more than just the highlights and top points and delve deeper into the details of the subject matter. This method might not help you in the cause and make it difficult for you to record more than just the highlights and headings. However, as mentioned earlier, you can get your way around this by making use of signs, symbols and acronyms to make it easier to record the information.

Sometimes, you might find that the notes you have made are not cohesive at all and do not make much sense. This indicates that you did not make the notes while being actively present in the moment and simply took down information that made sense to you in the spur of the moment.

You should bear in mind that being active and alert is one of the requisites of taking down notes. You should be present in the current moment so that you can make sense of what you are reading and write it down.

Some complain that this method makes it difficult to find information that is buried in between all the information that is recorded. However, there is a way around this as all you should do is add in headings and link them to a TOC. That way, you can easily go directly to the chosen place and read up on the information you need.

Remember that there is no one proper way of note taking that applies to all. You must ensure that you choose the one that suits you best. Do not listen to others and what they have to say about your note taking methods. If it works for you, then well and good, you can stick with it and make the most of your note taking habit.

Note Taking Methods

As you know, note taking is not a new trend and has existed since time immemorial. Note taking is a type of activity that is meant to help people reduce the effort put into understanding and recording the information. So, in effect, it helps people organize their data for easy reference.

Humans have been writing as long as language has existed and continue to write. Almost every aspect of writing has changed and, with it, note taking. People have completely changed the way in which notes are taken down, making it more efficient and easy.

In this segment, we look at some note taking techniques that you can use it to take down notes and make the most of your note taking habit.

The Cornell Method

The Cornell method for taking notes is quite popular and has been in existence for some time now. It is popular among students and is used widely. This method calls for sectioning off each page using different margins. So, instead of using the margin on the page, all you must do is draw lines at the bottom of the page. You can draw two more lines on top for the heading. You have to draw two on either side as well.

The segment at the bottom of the page will be kept for a summary of the page, where you write down the main points that were discussed in it. If you do not wish to highlight page-wise, then you can mention everything on the very last page and summarize the whole document. The approach you take up will depend on you and whatever you are comfortable with.

The section on top will be dedicated to the title of the page. Here is where you will write down a concise title that will tell you what the article is all about. You must leave about 3 inches space from the top of the margin. Some people find that this segment is unnecessary for all the pages and is good enough for just the front page. However, it is best to have this on top so that you know what the note is all about.

The side columns will be used for headings. As you begin writing in the body, you will start filling out the headings on the side. A majority of the information will be recorded in the body, and the headings will go on the side. These will act like subheadings and tell you what the body of the content contains. You can also add in any last minute information here so that you can refer back to it as and when you like.

Pros and cons

Like any other method, the Cornell comes with its share of pros and cons that are discussed as follows.

The Cornell note taking method is quite good for those who wish to keep their notes organized. Having the different columns all around helps students keep their notes neat and organized. Note taking, and understanding can help you concisely record information. You can write more and, more importantly, remember more.

This method can do wonders if you wish to take notes straight from a textbook. You can easily record all the information and highlight all the significant bits. You will find it much easier to use this method if you have the habit of using headings and subheadings while making notes.

The downside of this method is that you might have to review, then spend some time getting used to this method. Not everyone will be used to drawing lines on paper and might find tough to adjust to this new trend. You have to dedicate some time on a day to day to basis to practice this method. This might be a little difficult if you happen to be a fulltime student. You might also find it difficult to stick with this method if you are used to another method of taking notes.

One aspect to bear in mind while following this technique is that you have to pay close attention to what your lecturer is saying to be able to record all the information in an orderly fashion. You therefore have to get as much information as you can while taking down the notes.

If you wish to carry your laptop and record the information on it, then you must prepare the grid in advance so that you can record the information in it.

You can also consider recording the information in a regular format and then transfer it to a structured page. This might, however, turn out to be quite a time-consuming affair.

The Split-Page Method

The next method is known as the split page method of note taking. This type if quite similar to the previous one. Although they might appear to be similar, they have quite a few differences.

To use this method, all you do is split the page in half and use the left side for main ideas and the right side for secondary ideas. These will be those that will not be independent and depend on the primary ideas.

The best and easiest way to incorporate this method is by folding the page in half so that you create a central line between and write down the ideas on either side.

Pros and cons

Just as in the case of the Cornell method, this one comes with its share of pros and cons.

The advantage of this method is that it will help you organize all the data efficiently. You do not have to worry about your data being strewn all over the place. It will all be in one place thereby helping you access it easily.

The advantage that this method has over the Cornell method is that it is less time consuming and can be used by just about anyone to gather and record their thoughts. You do not have to whip out your pen and scale every time to draw the segments on the top, bottom and sides. You simply fold the paper, and your job will be done. If you want to make the line a little more prominent, then you can use a pen to draw over it.

The downside of this method is that, like the Cornell method, you have to pay close attention to what the lecturer is saying. If you do not, then you might end up missing out on important points. You will also find it time-consuming to divide the data into important and non-important points. There might also be a lack of space to add the headings.

Visual Aids

For those who are visual learners, there is a method that can be used. You will be able to create mind maps, graphs and other tables to make a connection and learn new things that are different from just the words on the page.

Some people find it that making use of this method greatly helps them as it is quite different and allows them to step away from regular note taking. So, for some, this method can work quite well owing to the way in which they learn things. It will also break the monotony and keep them from writing constantly.

Pros and cons

This method too has its set of pros and cons. As you know, this method only makes use of visual aid. This means that you might not be able to record all the information and find it difficult to put everything on paper. Therefore, you cannot consider this as your only method of taking notes. However, this method is quite amazing as it helps you take down more and remember things for longer. When you happen to be learning about systems and equations, you can make use of visual aids to help you learn better. You can not only learn more but also be able to recall everything easily.

Another advantage associated with this method is that it helps those who are unable to understand writing and rely wholly on visual aid for help. They can make use of this method to learn more and faster.

Shorthand Note taking

The shorthand method is a unique method to adopt. According to this method, all you are doing is using your own thing. This means that you put together two or more of the methods that you read on above to come up with a method of your own. That way, you can satisfy your intellectual needs.

When you make use of this method, you will have to be a little careful that you do not move away from the main point or complicate it for yourself. If you end up doing so, then you will be wasting your time spending too much time on one aspect.

Pros and cons

The advantage associated with this method is that you are allowed to make your own rules. There are no guidelines that you have to adhere to and you can go about setting your own guidelines. You can create the template yourself and use it as an outline. But remember, as mentioned earlier, it is possible for you to go into depths and details and become over picky about the material. So, keep in mind the method to follow and ensure that you choose a method that suits you best.

Annotation

Annotation is a method that is good for those who wish to use PowerPoint presentations or a note template that your professor might hand out to you. It consists of adding your notes and comments as the lecturer speaks. You can write down all the important notes down.

Many find this method useful as they can save paper, time and energy. These might prove to be expensive for a student, who can instead opt for tablets. It will be a one-time investment, and you can make as many notes as you like.

Pros and cons

Like other methods, this too has its share of ups and downs. The disadvantage associated with this method is that if your teacher does not give you notes before class, then you will find it a little difficult to take up this method. So, it will be detrimental to get the slides before each session for this method to work well.

Other Methods for Taking Notes

There are many other methods for taking notes. If you wish to know which ones then all you have to do is conduct a simple search and you will be able to find the different methods that can be taken up.

Some of the methods that are outlined are shorthand handwriting, which we mentioned earlier. You have to remember that when you wish to change the style, it can be a bit difficult and slow at first. But as and when you get used to it, you will be able to adapt to it in a better way.

Tips to take notes from books

When you take notes from a textbook, you have to keep many things in mind so that you do not end up wasting your time while taking down the notes. You will have to bear in mind a few things and practice them to make it easier to take notes.

The very first thing that you must do is read the book. This means that before you start taking notes or highlighting, you must read the page, paragraph, etc. This will make it easier for you to make the notes, as you will know what to emphasize and take down. If you jump into taking the notes without reading, then you might end up scratching out too many things.

You can make use of the Cornell method if you like so that you can easily take down all the information.

One easy way to make use of the Ryan Holiday method of note taking is to make use of sticky notes. You can replace the index cards with them and stick them on top of the page. That way, you will be able to save time and write down the cues quickly. All you have to do is look at the heading or subheading and know precisely what is on the page.

This will save you time, effort and make sure you find it easy to go through the notes and recall important information.

You can make use of a color-coding system using papers of a color for each chapter etc. This will make it even easier for you to find the information faster. Once you are done reading or wish to revise, then you can simply remove the note from the top and stick it back in its place.

When you take notes from a textbook, make sure that you are actively reading through. The more you read while writing, the easier it is for you to take notes. You will have the advantage of revising as you read. You will be able to absorb more information and retain it as well.

As and when you start going about picking notes from your textbook, your selective thinking pattern will kick in and make it easier for you to take down the notes. You will not have to think as much and will be able to pick out the crucial bits successfully.

If you wish to make it simple and fast, then all you must do is quickly go through the data and use a highlighter to highlight the important bits. You can then transfer the highlighted bits into your notebook. This will be simpler and faster. You will also be able to revise what you read.

As you can see, it is quite easy to transfer data from a textbook into your notebook. All you have to do is spend a little time picking out the essential bits and recording them one by one in your notebook or laptop.

Conclusion

With that, we have come to an end of this book. I thank you once again for choosing this book.

Do you still believe that notes are just notes? Hopefully, not! We have seen that notes are not just some facts on a piece of paper to review later, so we can get a good grade on the exam. Note taking is a learning tool. By thinking consciously about how we take notes and how to improve the quality of them, it can lead to good study practices and effective, long-term learning.

Successful people are good note takers and good note reviewers. Don't just take notes but review them frequently. Don't just read the notes, but interact with them. Test yourself on the notes, elaborate, comment, and complete them. Make recall hard if you want to make your memories last. Index your notes and refer back to them. Keep them organized, and they will save you lots of time and effort. Notes can do so many good things for you. They hold all your learning efforts. Treat them well. Look after them. Love your notes!

A final note!!!

I'm passionate about researching and discovering how we can optimally learn and make the most of life. I'm even more passionate about sharing all my experiences and connecting with you because this is how we'll all get better together. For this reason, please feel free to share your feedback and subscribe to my blog www.livediversified.com. I'm looking forward to hearing from you!

Go take some notes now! :)

***** Hey!!! Don't forget to download The Notetaker's Manifesto, a one-page PDF with all the good note-taking practices of this book!

To download, use this short link I have created http://bit.ly/2zsmP9C

*****

References

(1) Kiewra et al 1991.

(2) Hartley, James, and Alan Cameron∗. "Some observations on the efficiency of lecturing." *Educational Review* 20.1 (1967): 30-37.

(3) Locke, Edwin A. "An empirical study of lecture note taking among college students." *The journal of educational research* 71.2 (1977): 93-99.

(4) Johnstone, Alex H., and WY Su. "Lectures-a learning experience?." *EDUCATION IN CHEMISTRY-LONDON-* 31.3 (1994): 75-75.

(5) Piolat, Annie, Thierry Olive, and Ronald T. Kellogg. "Cognitive effort during note taking." *Applied Cognitive Psychology* 19.3 (2005): 291-312.

* * *

Notes on Note-Taking: Review of Research and Insights for Students and Instructors. Michael C. Friedman. Harvard Initiative for Learning and Teaching. Harvard University.

Research on Student Note Taking: Implications for Faculty and Graduate Student Instructors. Center for Research on Learning and Teaching. Deborah DeZure, Matthew Kaplan, Martha Deerman.

Kiewra, K. A. (1987). Note taking and review: The research and its implications. Journal of Instructional Science, 16, 233-249.

Hartley, J. (2002). Notetaking in non-academic settings: A review. Applied Cognitive Psychology, 16, 559–574. doi:10.1002/acp.814.

Bjork, R. A., & Allen, T. W. (1970). The spacing effect: Consolidation or differential encoding? Journal of Verbal Learning and Verbal Behavior, 9, 567-572.

Bjork, R. A., Dunlosky, J., & Kornell, N. (2013). Self-regulated learning: Beliefs, techniques, and illusions. Annual Review of Psychology, 64, 417-444.

Piolat, A., Olive, T., & Kellogg, R. T. (2005). Cognitive effort during note taking. Applied Cognitive Psychology, 19, 291-312.

Muller, P. A., & Oppenheimer, D. M. (in press). The pen is mightier than the keyboard: Advantages of longhand over laptop note taking. Psychological Science.

Peper, R. J., & Mayer, R. E. (1978). Note taking as a generative activity. Journal of Educational Psychology, 70, 514-522.

Van der Meer, J. (2012). Students' note-taking challenges in the twenty-first century: Considerations for teachers and academic staff developers. Teaching in Higher Education, 17, 13–23. doi:10.1080/13562517.2011.590974.

Internet Links

The Note-taker's Manifesto http://bit.ly/2zsmP9C

Cornell note-taking system
(http://lsc.cornell.edu/LSC_Resources/cornellsystem.pdf)

YouTube video (about the Cornell note-taking system)
(www.youtube.com/watch?v=4vOsVKWeyAA)

link to abbreviations
(www.adelaide.edu.au/writingcentre/learning_guides/learningGuide_note-takingAbbreviations.pdf)

The 4-Hour Workweek by Tim Ferriss (http://fourhourworkweek.com)

tips by Tim Ferriss (http://fourhourworkweek.com/2007/12/05/how-to-take-notes-like-an-alpha-geek-plus-my-2600-date-challenge/)

recent study proves that taking notes by hand promotes long-term recall
(http://pss.sagepub.com/content/early/2014/04/22/0956797614524581.abstract)

Another study that used advanced techniques like electromagnetic resonance has shown that handwriting activates regions of the brain associated with thinking, language, and memory.
(http://www.wsj.com/articles/SB10001424052748704631504575531932754922518)

Connect with the Author

Other books by Angelos Georgakis:

Learn Russian Diversified (http://livediversified.com/books/learn-russian-diversified/)

The Superlearner Myth (http://livediversified.com/books/the-superlearner-myth/)

How to Learn a Language NOT in Seven Days (http://livediversified.com/books/how-to-learn-any-language-not-in-7-days/)

* * *

Connect with me:

E-mail: livediversified@gmail.com

Follow me on Twitter: https://twitter.com/angelosgeo

Friend me on Facebook: http://facebook.com/angelos.georgakis

Follow me on YouTube:
https://www.youtube.com/c/AngelosGeorgakis

Subscribe to my blog: http://livediversified.com

* * *

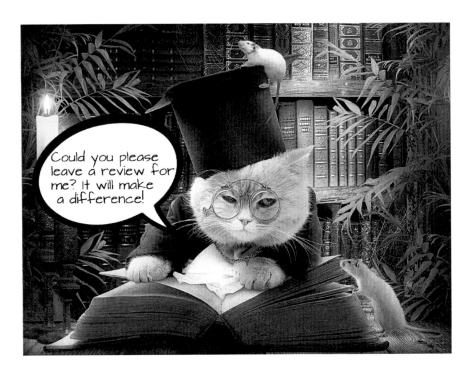

If you enjoyed this book, then I'd like to ask you for a favor. Would you be kind enough to leave a review for this book on Amazon or Goodreads (www.goodreads.com)?

Thanks!
Angelos Georgakis

Made in the USA
Middletown, DE
28 December 2017